M000223854

CELIAC DISEASE

SAFE/UNSAFE FOOD LIST AND ESSENTIAL INFORMATION ON LIVING WITH A GLUTEN FREE DIET

Also by Jaqui Karr:

"Solace from depression"

A book that is a place of solace, support, understanding, and compassion - balanced with nutritional information that is relevant and immediately applicable. Besides the difficulties of life in general, our environment can make us truly ill or weaken our system to a point that makes it a challenge to cope. Learn how your health can be immediately improved. You can't beat something that you don't understand. Learn how to nourish your body properly and naturally so that you can give yourself the strength and physiological advantage to win.

"Gratitude is the Answer; the Secret to Happiness"

We have all had journals throughout the years, but it seems we write in them only when we are feeling good and have good things to write. In reality, we need inspiration more during times that we aren't feeling so great. This one is designed to help you through those challenging days, the days that you need a little help in changing your mood and mind frame. The author has shared parts of her own journal with you in the hope that perhaps a thought or a single word will help connect you to something you have become disconnected from, perhaps discover joy and pleasure from something you never noticed before. A unique journal that offers you the little nudge you might need to open your heart and mind to a place of serenity, beauty, gratitude...freedom...

Available from Amazon.com and other fine retailers worldwide

"This book is a must-have for anyone living with Celiac Disease. It contains a wealth of extremely valuable information, unknown to most health care practitioners. This book is filled with tips and tricks that can help patients avoid a great deal of pain and suffering. It is also a useful gift for friends and family of Celiac sufferers as it can help them understand the complexity and repercussions of the disease."

Dr. A. Lepage-Chaumont, N.D.
Pure Med Naturopathic Centre

NO
TWO
CELIACS

ARE EXACTLY THE SAME

Being a certified nutritionist, natural health consultant, as well as a Celiac myself, I have created this reference book to provide a practical on-hand guide to help manage a gluten free diet.

This guide provides the most complete and accurate list of safe and unsafe ingredients found in commercial products, where to look for hidden dangers, and why some common ingredients shown as safe on many gluten free lists are not necessarily always safe. You will also find several items that you will not see on most other lists, and crucial processing and packaging information that affect the safety of things we consume daily.

As a health consultant, I felt it important to also point out certain products - even though gluten free, that have been proven as toxic, yet are still legal. These have been indicated for your consideration.

This book is listed by ingredient, not final product, so that it is always current and relevant to you, regardless of geographic location, as well as when manufacturers change an ingredient (which is often). The advantage to you is to have a resource that is constant, a reliable reference that will always help you choose the right foods.

The slim, pocketbook format makes it easy to keep on hand and makes it convenient to carry with you when grocery shopping or traveling. Also, additional space is included to add items based on your individual reaction to specific foods or beverages.

The reality is that NO TWO CELIACS ARE ALIKE – this might be the most significant thing for any Celiac to remember. It means that besides the basic list of foods we all know we definitely cannot eat, there will be varied reactions to many other food items. Due to that fact, this list, or any other, can *never* be absolute.

It is important that you add your own list of what does not agree with your body. There are several blank pages at the back of this guide for you to keep track of any foods that don't work well with you. This will help you customize and keep this crucially important list all in one place, and keep you safe.

Please read the entire front section thoroughly – it is written in a concise, summarized way to make it easy to read quickly and it truly *is* ESSENTIAL information, including a specific vitamin and mineral list for Celiacs, particularly when newly diagnosed.

Managing a condition that imposes limitations on so many foods can be challenging, but like anything new, being well informed and having the proper tools makes all the difference.

I trust you will find this guide to be an invaluable tool and hope some words of encouragement from one Celiac to another provides you some comfort. In time, you will see that being a Celiac is actually quite a blessing; it provides wholesome eating habits, which in turn provides for much greater health.

I wish you infinite health and wellness.

Jaqui Karr, C.S.N.

NakedFood.ca

CONTENTS

ESSENTIAL BASICS

ARTIFICIAL FLAVOR/COLOR: always side with caution when you see vague or general terms. Food coloring can contain many ingredients within itself. Artificial flavors and colors may or may not be safe; only the manufacturer can confirm if they used any ingredients containing gluten.

CANDY, CHOCOLATE, COUGH DROPS: almost always dusted with flour to prevent sticking, and since the flour is not an actual ingredient IN the candy, the manufacturer usually will not list it. Today there are so many gluten free versions of these products available, it is quite easy to substitute. Look for specific labeling indicating gluten free.

CHEESE: most cheeses are safe, but not all. Blue cheese, Chilton, Roquefort are not safe; avoid veined cheeses or any that are coated with "mystery" products. Mystery products almost always contain gluten. Also avoid pre-shredded cheeses; they can be dusted with flour to prevent sticking. As with anything else you consume, check each ingredient on the label since recipes can vary.

COLAS & COMMON DRINKS: many of them are gluten free but caution with caramel coloring, it is an ingredient made up of several others, and the recipes vary. Be on alert with root beers, and any specially flavored drinks – the honey colored drinks should raise a flag. Distilled alcohol is generally safe, though vodka & rum manufacturers outright state their flavored vodkas are not safe for Celiacs. Wine coolers and regular beer are definitely unsafe, but there are GF versions available. Wine is safe (both red and white), as are champagne, port, and sherry.

CROSS-CONTAMINATION

Eating at a friend's or even hosting your own party, some simple precautions will go a long way. Double dipping can be a catastrophe. Ask your host to put aside a little plate with a spoon or two of dips before any guests arrive – this will ensure that no one with regular crackers or chips will contaminate food that you might also consume. Same rule applies to cheese; cut a few pieces of safe cheeses for yourself before substances from unsafe cheeses contaminate through the knives or platter. Avoid touching the bread basket when it is passed around – the flour dust can transfer easily to your hands. And please don't ever feel bad - you would happily accommodate anyone with a food intolerance and your friends will feel the same way.

When dining out, good humor and asking politely will certainly go a long way, but be sure you are clear about the severity of your gluten intolerance. Your health is ultimately your responsibility. Let's take a safe item like potatoes – if you are ordering fries, find out if other items, like breaded onion rings, are cooked in the same fryer. If so, then the oil will be contaminated. Whether eating out or at a friend's, never be shy to ask questions about preparation, seasoning, cooking tools. Consider things like gravy (usually thickened with flour). Take time to consider typical toppings or side dishes that may make an otherwise safe dish, unsafe.

For store bought foods, check every ingredient and when in doubt, contact the manufacturer. This is particularly important with ingredients that can be made from several sources, like maltodextrin. Also be cautious with ingredients within ingredients like vinegar in mayonnaise: the particular vinegar the manufacturer used may or may not be safe.

DETOX & DIETS: please proceed with caution and consult with your doctor. Any kind of diet, especially a restrictive one such as a diet with no fruit allowed, can create nutritional deficiencies (which is true for *any*one, Celiac or not). Good health comes from plenty of wholesome foods of a wide variety.

If you absolutely feel the need for a cleanse, consult with a knowledgeable, certified professional to guide you through a juice fast that includes plenty of nutrients. Avoid colon cleanses within first year of diagnoses as this will wash away minerals from your body at a time when you need to be restoring them.

A word about nutritionists: as much as they might mean well, there are very few who understand Celiac well. Be sure that their certification does not misguide you. Celiac is complex and should never be compared to standard diets or allergies.

GLUTEN FREE AND WHEAT FREE ARE NOT THE SAME: gluten comes in many forms (page 24) – check individual ingredients. "Wheat free" alone is not safe.

GRAS (GENERALLY RECOGNIZED AS SAFE): caution with the term "harmless level of gluten". Gastroenterologists with extensive Celiac experience will tell you there is no such thing as a harmless level of gluten to a Celiac. The only prudent way to handle this disease is to remain 100% gluten free.

GROCERY GUIDES: can misguide you because manufacturers regularly change their ingredients. Numerous items that were safe at the time the guide was published might not be safe just months later. By law, labels must always be changed when ingredients change, so the only truly safe route is to always check every ingredient on every label.

GROUND SPICE: buy spices in their whole form and grind at home (this also tastes so much better). Inexpensive grinders make it so simple. Besides the fact that pre-ground spices comprise risks of cross contamination, you might also be consuming harmful toxins. I.e. many table salts are bleached for a brighter white color; this is done with a harmful chemical that goes unnoticed since we consume salt in small doses. Good salt options are pure Himalayan or gray sea salt, it may cost you an extra few dollars a year – this is such a nominal amount, yet the cumulative effect of several minor changes will be significant.

KITCHEN CARE:

Get two cutting boards and make sure they are different materials to avoid mix-ups or residual matter; glass for gluten free and wood for standard (wood tends to trap substance even after washed).

Keep the standard food, utensils, toaster, on bottom shelves to keep crumbs from falling onto gluten free shelves. Same for refrigerator and cupboards – dedicate the top shelves for gluten free items.

Do not wipe crumbs from counters with the same hand or tea towels that you might use to dry plates.

Use different colored containers to store gluten free food. Keep two sets of colors to avoid mix-ups.

Tape "GF" stickers onto peanut butter jars, butter, and all other foods prone to double dipping or spreading onto bread; dedicate one set to remain gluten free.

-*Do not be discouraged,* these are all things that need to be set up just once, soon they will be second nature for you and your family.

MEDICATION: our focus is usually on food alone, especially when newly diagnosed, but *EVERY* single thing we digest must be checked. Unfortunately, your doctor will usually not know which medication is gluten free – but pharmacists can find out for you.

MINDSET: no different from everything else in life, your attitude towards this whole adventure will make all the difference in the world. Notice the reference to it as an adventure and not anything restrictive. If you moved to a foreign country and did not have access to the foods you are used to, you would undoubtedly adjust and enjoy new tastes. This is an opportunity for you to discover new foods and great new recipes.

MODIFIED – *ANYTHING*: unless you are 100% certain it is pure corn starch, it is unsafe. The term "modified food" or "modified x product" is very vague and unsafe. "Modified" can mean anything.

NATURAL FLAVOR & COLOR: Do not let the word "natural" misguide you; *wheat is a natural product...* Always be careful with vague and general terms.

NON-FOOD ITEMS: Cosmetics (particularly lipstick, lip balm) chewing gum, breath mints, toothpaste, mouthwash, envelopes, stamps, (buy self-sealing); look at everything you will digest with a sharper eye, and when in doubt – avoid or replace it.

RAW: of course going raw will ensure absolute safety, but it is not easy or convenient for most people. Even if not a completely raw diet, try to go to raw forms with as much as possible: i.e. homemade pesto instead of from a jar. You can't imagine how much better homemade salad dressings taste, and most will keep for over a week.

SAFE FOODS: be aware of seasoning, coloring, flavoring, marinades. The obvious may be simple: "avoid breaded chicken". Watch for the not-so-obvious like wheat in ice cream, barley in sauces and dressings, malt in chocolate, wheat in soy sauce...check ALL the ingredients in everything you consume.

SUSHI: very high risk of cross contamination with breaded, fried, tempura foods. There is also a major health concern outside of gluten; it is best explained in the extraordinary documentary "The Cove". "Mercury Rising" in the special features section discusses concerns with sushi; *highly recommended* to view this movie for health as well as environmental concerns.

TEA: many contain unsafe flavoring products, check labels carefully. There is a risk of cross contamination during the packaging process since most tea producers offer varieties of flavors. Teas are also an item where vague terms such as "natural flavors" are found often. Whenever possible, buy whole leaf teas.

THE LAW: most countries' laws state that an ingredient does not have to be listed if the product contains less than 100 grams (amount varies) per kilo or less than a certain number ppm (parts per million). ANY amount of gluten, no matter how little, is harmful to a Celiac. Please look out for petitions you can sign to help groups trying to get the government to change these dangerous laws; consumers have a right to know exactly what is in any product they buy.

VINEGAR: apple cider, distilled, wine, balsamic are usually safe. White vinegar might not be; the manufacturer can use wheat, rye or barley in their process and non-distilled contains gluten. If you do not have clear information, avoid it. Very inexpensive white vinegar should raise an alert flag and be verified.

VITAMIN DEFICIENCIES: Deficiencies caused by all autoimmune disorders are a very severe matter and can cause numerous complications including fatigue, depression, and other physical issues. If you have a gastroenterologist who knows Celiac well, by all means, work closely with them. You may also want to consult with a nutritionist to evaluate your diet, help you with substitutions to suit your lifestyle, as well as provide insight with whether or not you are consuming enough nutrients or require supplements.

Please be sure to confirm if your nutritionist thoroughly understands gluten intolerance. Also depending on how long you went undiagnosed (average Celiac goes undiagnosed for 11 years), your system may be in a serious state of deficiency and you will require special supplementation until you have restored what is necessary (essentials on next page).

VITAMINS & SUPPLEMENTS: Many contain fillers, binders, coloring, and/or flavoring. Always check all ingredients as you do with food.

Take whatever you can find in liquid or lozenge form; these are assimilated into your body more easily.

Without a doubt take enteric coated superior probiotics daily. You want enteric coated because you want the live acidophilus cells to reach your intestines intact – when they are not enteric coated, over 90% of their potency is lost with the natural acids in your stomach.

IMPORTANT TO NOTE: Supplementing may be necessary at first to restore your health and balance - avoid using supplements as a lifelong replacement for a balanced healthy diet. Ideally you want to be getting all your nutrients from organic foods in your daily diet.

ESSENTIAL VITAMINS: the following 4 pages will list the essential vitamins you need and some guidance on determining dosages. Celiac is complex and can cause a lot of complications that you can completely prevent, and many you can reverse. Cross check this list with your diet: i.e. if you drink pure orange juice, eat kiwis or strawberries daily, you don't need vitamin C supplements. Note there are many more benefits than listed here, details summarized to our focus.

Vitamins A and E: heal & repair the intestinal tract. A: 600-800 micrograms/day. E: 400-600 IU/day.

B Complex: energy and proper digestion. If it does not contain at least 100mcg of **B6** and **B12 each**, take them in addition to the B Complex.

Folic Acid (called folate when from food): needed for protein metabolism, memory, fights depression. Critically important for pregnant women. 1mg/day.

Calcium, Vitamin D, Magnesium: listed together because you can usually find them in one pill or bottle, and because you absorb them better when taken together. Celiacs are very commonly deficient in all 3 of these. Vitamin D tells your body to absorb calcium as well as helps fight depression; most of us are not absorbing D from the 15-20 minutes of direct sun we need daily and need to supplement. New studies are also showing D as a preventative vitamin to MS and so much more. Calcium is critical for bone strength (exercise also important for this). Take soluble versions for better absorption: calcium citrate, lactate, or gluconate (not carbonate). Magnesium is also essential for bone health, proper function of muscles & nerves, and helps your body absorb calcium. Calcium & magnesium together help maintain normal pH value in the body.

Vitamin C: 250mg/day. This will strengthen your immune system, decrease stress and blood pressure, and cause your body to secrete lower levels of cortisol (stress hormone). WARNING: vitamin C boosts absorption of iron, which your body can not eliminate from your system (when in excess). Never take iron supplements without professional guidance.

Vitamin K: most Celiacs show a deficiency of this vitamin, which can lead to blood clotting. A superior multi-vitamin should contain the 10mcg needed.

Potassium: third most abundant mineral in the body, and commonly a deficiency in Celiacs. Eat a kiwi, banana, or potato 4-5 times/week. Kiwi is a superfood for many vitamins, daily intake is recommended.

Omega 3 Fatty Acids: vital for brain and nerve function. DHA helps brain cells communicate with each other, restore chemical balance, and prevent nerve abnormalities. Taken with B6, B12, and folate – it is an essential anti-depressant formula. DHA is formed with the correct ratio of omega 3 and 6. Best sources are krill oil & fish oil; absolutely critical to verify that you are buying mercury/cadmium/lead free products. 1000-2000mg/day.

Flax Seed Oil: A super oil containing omega 3's, 6's and 9's, B vitamins, potassium, lecithin, magnesium, fiber, protein, zinc, and 100 times richer in lignin than most whole grains. Incredibly long list of benefits, some of which are to reduce risk of breast & colon cancer, lower cholesterol, prevent blood clots, increase your own body's energy production and muscle recovery, stimulates brown fat cells facilitating weight loss, improves liver function, and can even treat some cases of depression. Everyone, Celiac or not, should be taking a minimum of 1000mg/day.

DETERMINING DOSAGES: the key element regarding dosages is that one size never fits all. Every person needs a customized formula based on their individual needs, and those needs will keep changing with age, changes in diet, activity level, and variations in health status.

The RDA (recommended dietary allowances) found on most products is usually far too low. RDA's were created decades ago to keep people alive by preventing diseases like scurvy. They were not created to provide optimal health and certainly are not current to the needs we face today due to diminished nutritional value and increased toxic value of our foods and water.

Unless you have blood tests showing deficiencies with particular items, you will need to do a little experimenting to see what works for you (of course, best option always is to coordinate with a professional). If you are managing supplements on your own, first thing to know is the difference between water and fat soluble vitamins.

Water soluble means your body can easily excrete what it doesn't need through your urine and sweat, so you don't need to worry about taking too much (within reason of course, 40,000mg of anything is harmful). Fat soluble means your body stores excess amounts in fats through your bloodstream; really excessive amounts can become toxic, but it takes very high amounts to get there. It is always best to consult with a qualified health care provider.

WATER SOLUBLE: all B vitamins, including folic acid, and vitamin C

FAT SOLUBLE: vitamins A, D, E, K

If you do consume a little too much in fat soluble, long before it gets to any toxic or dangerous level, you will feel yourself getting a little tired and lethargic – this is your body telling you there is too much for it to process. The trick is to go ahead with water soluble vitamins, and then with the fat soluble ones, start with RDA's and then one by one, increase dosages in small increments and see how you feel. This will take several months to accomplish because you need to isolate each fat soluble vitamin for 2-3 weeks as you try different levels. You must do this one at a time so that you know exactly how you are reacting to each particular vitamin.

When you start this process, your body might be quite depleted of certain vitamins and you will need higher amounts before you can bring it back down. For example, you may need 3000 IU/day of vitamin D for months before your system has stored enough to be at optimal level. Once your body is stable with correct stores, 600-1000 IU/day is sufficient. Do not be afraid when incrementing in small amounts.

What can be harmful in excessive amounts are iron, zinc, copper...these are easy to identify – they are the metals. And you'll notice they are not in the "essential vitamins" listed in this book. It is not recommended and can be harmful to experiment with metals without the guidance of a physician.

With fish oils or omega fatty acids, make sure you are buying a brand certified free of chemicals and metals (mercury, cadmium, lead). The optimum is to find a brand that uses an independent lab to test purity.

If you are fighting depression, the key elements are folic acid, B vitamins, and omega-3's (DHA/EPA).

The Discrepancies

As information is flooded in from various sources, you may find a lot of conflicting data. Foods listed as unsafe on some lists will be listed as safe on others and it can be very frustrating. There are many reasons this happens, one of which is that Celiac is not a black and white condition. Another main issue is that our small world shares much of its food in imports and exports, but there is no standard as far as labeling or process.

Even products all scientists agree to be safe may not be because when researchers experiment in a contained laboratory, they find the product to be safe. The reality is, several of those products, like quinoa and buckwheat, are often contaminated because they are processed and packaged in plants that also process regular wheat. If you visit one of these facilities and see the flour dust everywhere (looks like a snow blizzard in Canada, employees are walking around in astronaut suits), it becomes clear why anything else processed in that plant will be contaminated. These items have been marked with comments to help you proceed with caution, look for 100% GF facilities.

Some foods, like maltodextrin, can be made from wheat, potato, corn, or other starches. Known instances of this have been indicated; for these items, the manufacturer must clarify which product it used.

As well, different countries use different ingredients for the same food. An example is MSG: in the U.S. it is usually made with corn, outside the U.S. it is made with wheat or soy. If the testing lab used a soy based product and listed it as safe, but you consume the wheat version...this is also where many gluten free food guides go wrong.

It is frustrating to see "confirm with manufacturer" when you are expecting a list to tell you what is safe or unsafe. The reality is, NO list can truthfully claim to provide accurate information on every item – it's simply not possible. At best, a list can confirm most items, and indicate caution for indeterminate ones.

Whenever you are in doubt or a food listed as safe still seems to affect you in a negative way, keep track of it in your personal notes and completely avoid the food. Discuss these items with your doctor, they might be able to make a connection to other allergies or factors common to Celiacs.

Many Celiacs tend to develop food allergies apart from their gluten intolerance, like lactose intolerance or nut allergies. If you are on a completely gluten free diet yet still feel pain or even discomfort, ask your doctor for food allergy tests. It seems quite unfair for further allergies to be a side effect when we are already restricted to so many foods – but the reality is there are such worse illnesses out there, let's be grateful that ours can be managed through diet alone.

Fortunately, there are more and more new gluten free products coming onto the market; just be careful as government GF standards are not absolute – this guide will help identify potential areas of danger.

Food intolerances are rising at an alarming rate and will continue to rise until consumer demands force manufacturers to stop adding toxins to all our foods. In time, with heightened awareness and consumer pressure, the food industry will be forced to respond.

All of this may feel quite overwhelming at first, but it is critical information that will help you manage your new diet. *You'll have a handle on this before you know it.*

GRAINS AND GLUTEN

There are a handful of studies going back more than 20 years showing Celiac patients reacting to rice and/or corn yet most government agencies and medical communities are accepting corn and rice as safe. Most communities, *but not all.*

I know many of us rely heavily on rice when we eliminate other glutens from our diets, so yet another restriction is not welcome news.

If you have been gluten free for more than 6 months and still not feeling quite back to 100%, even if it is not full blown symptoms, perhaps eliminating rice and corn for 1-6 months would be a good experiment. If you find yourself feeling completely fantastic after a while, then you will know for yourself. I have listed them as unsafe in this guide because there are conflicting reports and we can't say with complete certainty that they are safe. Perhaps there are variables that differ from one Celiac to another so while one may tolerate these grains well, another may not. Those variables are far from being discovered. Right now the focus is on methods of testing, looking for certain genes, etc.

As it stands, I don't think the medical community will be presenting a unanimous decision anytime soon, if ever, so it will remain up to each individual to make a choice. We don't know yet what the long term effects of continuous digestion of small amounts of gluten are and we know that in most cases the person will be suffering internal damage with no external symptoms.

This one will come down to individual decisions; sadly the burden sits with you, the patient.

The most controversial discrepancy: corn and rice are "known" as safe yet all grains have gluten. The reason some have been labeled as safe is due to the lower levels of gluten or lower levels of glutamine. "Prolamins" are: proteins high in PROLine and glutAMINe. Gliadin and glutenin are the prolamins for wheat, and this being the highest percentage of gluten within grains has become the focus of most studies, but gliadin is not the only offender to Celiac Disease.

Barley (hordein 45-55%)
Corn (zein 55%)
Millet (panicin 20-40%)*
Oats (avenin 16%)
Rice (orzenin 5%)
Rye (secalin 30-50%)
Sorgum (kafirin 52%)
Wheat (gliadin/glutenin 69%)

*Millet may be a controversy within a controversy – some studies claim it has zero gluten because its prolamin is not "glutelin-like", particularly in the finger & foxtail varieties. These are generally older studies and not considering Celiac.

We know some patients react to corn, rice, and all other grains, but we don't know why others might not. Issues to consider:

1) The body's immediate reaction, or lack thereof, (even with those who react acutely with higher levels of gluten) is not a good measuring stick
2) We don't yet know what the long term implications of small amounts (as in rice) of gluten are. Please read the article posted at: Naked.Food.ca/legal.php

Again, due to the conflicting studies, rice, corn, and their by-products have been marked as unsafe in this guide – but ultimately the decision is yours.

GLUTEN FREE VERSIONS OF MANY UNSAFE PRODUCTS, LIKE BEERS AND CERTAIN CHEESES, ARE NOW AVAILABLE – your motto should always be "check every ingredient on every label"

SAFE & UNSAFE INGREDIENT LIST

☑safe ⊗unsafe ?caution or specifics needed

⊗Abyssinian Hard (wheat triticum durum)
☑Acacia Gum
☑Acesulfame K
☑Acesulfame Potassium
☑Acetanisole
☑Acetic Acid
☑Acetic Anhydride
☑Acetolactate Decarboxylase
☑Acetone
☑Acetone Peroxide
☑Acetophenone
⊗Acidophilus Milk
☑Acorn Quercus
☑Active Bacterial Cultures
☑Adipic Acid
☑Adzuki Bean
☑Agar
☑Agave
☑Alant Starch
☑Albumen
?Alcohol:

  SAFE: Distilled alcohol [unflavored gin, rum, vodka, whiskey], champagne, port, sherry, wine.

  NOT SAFE: Specially flavored rum, vodka, premixes, beer, wine coolers. Sake contains Koji, which may contain barley. Cider may contain barley enzymes.

  As with food, if all the ingredients haven't been verified or are unavailable, refrain until you can verify with manufacturer or find a gluten free substitute

⊗ Ale
☑ Alfalfa
☑ Algae
☑ Algin
☑ Alginate
☑ Alginic Acid
☑ Alkalized Cocoa
☑ Alkanet
☑ Allicin
☑ Allura Red
☑ Almond
☑ Alpha-amylase
☑ Alpha-lactalbumin
☑ Alpha-tocopherol Acetate
☑ Aluminum
☑ Amaranth (possible cross contamination)
☑ Ambergris
☑ Ammonium Alginate
☑ Ammonium Bicarbonate or Carbonate
☑ Ammonium Carrageenan
☑ Ammonium Chloride
☑ Ammonium Citrate
☑ Ammonium Furcelleran
☑ Ammonium Hydroxide
☑ Ammonium Persulphate
☑ Ammonium Phosphate
☑ Ammonium Sulphate
⊗ Amp-Isostearoyl Hydrolyzed Wheat Protein
☑ Amylase
☑ Amylopectin
☑ Amylose
☑ Anise

☑Annatto
? Annatto Color (multiple processing methods)
☑Anthocyanins
☑Apple Cider Vinegar
☑Arabic Gum
☑Arabinogalactan
⊗Arborio Rice (see page 24)
☑Arrowroot (pure arrowroot is safe; commercially prepared arrow biscuits usually contain gluten)
? Artificial Butter Flavor (recipes/ingredients vary)
? Artificial Color (vague)
? Artificial Flavor (vague)
⊗Asafoetida (spice, often contains flour)
☑Ascorbic Acid
☑Aspartame (gluten free, but highly toxic)
☑Aspartic Acid
☑Aspic
☑Astragalus Gummifer
⊗Atta Flour
☑Autolyzed Yeast Extract
⊗Avena Sativa (oats - see page 24)
⊗Avenin (see page 24)
☑Avidin
☑Azodicarbonamide (gluten free, but toxic)
☑Bacon (caution flavoring/spices)
☑Bacterial Cultures
? Baking Powder (verify which starch is used)
? Baking Soda (verify all ingredients, not all are safe)
☑Balsamic Vinegar
⊗Barley
⊗Barley Grass
⊗Barley Hordeum Vulgare
⊗Barley Malt

⊗ Basmati Rice (see page 24)
☑ Beans
⊗ Beer
☑ Beeswax
☑ Bengal Gram
☑ Benzoic Acid
☑ Benzoyl Peroxide
☑ Benzyl Alcohol
☑ Besan bean (chickpea)
☑ Beta Carotene
⊗ Beta Glucan (oats - see page 24)
☑ Betaine
☑ BHA
☑ BHT
☑ Bicarbonate of Soda
☑ Biotin
⊗ Black Rice (see page 24)
⊗ Bleached Flour
⊗ Blue Cheese (small amounts of flour in the mold)
⊗ Bouillon
☑ Bovine Rennet
⊗ Bran
⊗ Bread Flour
⊗ Brewer's Rice (see page 24)
⊗ Brewer's Yeast
⊗ Brie Cheese (caution with coating)
☑ Bromelain
☑ Brominated Vegetable Oil (gluten free, often in colas, toxic in high amounts and banned in many countries)
⊗ Broth (many GF versions available)
⊗ Brown Flour

⊗ Brown Rice Syrup (see page 24)
☑ Brown Sugar
☑ Buckwheat (risk of cross contamination)
⊗ Bulgur
☑ Butter (unflavored, check ingredients)
? Buttermilk (most contain modified food starch)
⊗ Butterscotch
☑ Butylated Hydroxyanisole
☑ Butylated Hydroxytoluene
☑ Butyl Compounds
☑ Caffeine
☑ Calcium Acetate
☑ Calcium Alginate
☑ Calcium Aluminum Silicate
☑ Calcium Ascorbate
☑ Calcium Carbonate
☑ Calcium Carrageenan
? Calcium Caseinate (contains MSG)
☑ Calcium Chloride
☑ Calcium Citrate
☑ Calcium Disodium
☑ Calcium Fumarate
☑ Calcium Furcelleran
☑ Calcium Gluconate
☑ Calcium Glycerophosphate
☑ Calcium Hydroxide
☑ Calcium Hypophosphite
☑ Calcium Iodate
☑ Calcium Lactate
☑ Calcium Pantothenate
☑ Calcium Peroxide
☑ Calcium Phosphate

☑Calcium Propionate
☑Calcium Silicate
☑Calcium Sorbate
☑Calcium Stearate
☑Calcium Stearoyl Lactylate
☑Calcium Sulfate
☑Calcium Tartrate
⊗Calrose Rice (see page 24)
⊗Camembert Cheese (caution with coating)
☑Camphor (gluten free, poisonous in large amounts)
?Candy (often dusted with flour to prevent sticking)
☑Cane Sugar
☑Cane Vinegar
☑Canola Oil (also called rapeseed oil. made from the seed of rape - which is in the grass family. tested as safe but many Celiacs have adverse reactions. Canola is a genetically modified product that your body doesn't process well)
☑Canthaxanthin
☑Caprylic Acid
?Caramel Color (often made with barley malt, manufacturer must confirm ingredients used)
☑Caraway Seeds
☑Carbonated Water
☑Carbon Dioxide
☑Carboxymethyl Cellulose
☑Carmine
☑Carnauba Wax
☑Carob Bean
☑Carob Bean Gum
☑Carob Flour
☑Carrageenan
☑Carrageenan Chondrus Crispus

☑Casein
☑Cassava Manihot Esculenta
☑Castor Oil
☑Catalase
☑Cellulase
☑Cellulose
☑Cellulose Ether
☑Cellulose Gum
⊗Cereal Binding
☑Cetyl Alcohol
☑Cetyl Stearyl Alcohol
☑Champagne Vinegar
☑Channa (chickpea)
☑Charcoal
❓Cheese (not all are safe, check the labels carefully; blue and veined cheese usually contain trace amounts of flour, also avoid pre-shredded cheeses as they are usually coated with flour to avoid sticking or clumping)
☑Chestnuts
☑Chia
☑Chicken (fresh is safe; caution with pre-seasoned)
☑Chickpea
⊗Chilton cheese
☑Chlorella
☑Chlorine
☑Chloropentafluoroethane
☑Chlorophyll
❓Chocolate (usually unsafe, also many bars are dusted with flour to avoid sticking to wrapping)
❓Chocolate Liquor (look for added ingredients)
☑Cholecalciferol
☑Choline Chloride

⊗Chorizo (usually contain cereal fillers, avoid if you don't have detailed label or verify with manufacturer)

⊗Chow Mein Noodles

☑Chromium Citrate

☑Chymosin

?Citric Acid (verify source used)

?Clarifying Agents (may be hydrolyzed wheat)

⊗Club Wheat (triticum aestivum subspecies compactum)

☑Cochineal

☑Cocoa (verify it is pure cocoa)

☑Cocoa Butter

☑Coconut

☑Coconut Flour

☑Coconut Oil

☑Coconut Vinegar

☑Coffee (pure coffee is safe, though many Celiacs are sensitive - careful with flavors added when buying lattes and cappuccinos, or flavored milk)

☑Collagen

☑Colloidal Silicon Dioxide

⊗Common Wheat (Triticum aestivum)

☑Confectioner's Glaze or Sugar

⊗Converted® Rice (see page 24)

?Cooking Spray (many contain grain or flour alcohol)

☑Copernicia Cerifera

☑Copper Sulphate

⊗Corn and all by-products (see page 24)

☑Cortisone

☑Cotton Seed

☑Cotton Seed Oil

⊗ Couscous
☑ Cowitch
☑ Cowpea
⊗ Cracker Meal
☑ Cream of Tartar (watch for added flavoring)
⊗ Criped Rice
☑ Crospovidone
⊗ Croutons
☑ Curcumin
☑ Curds
☑ Curry (pure curry safe; paste may contain gluten)
⊗ Custard
☑ Cyanocobalamin
☑ Cyclamate
☑ Cysteine, L
☑ Dal or Dahl (lentils)
☑ D-Alpha-tocopherol
☑ Dasheen Flour (taro)
☑ Dates (may be coated to prevent sticking)
☑ D-Calcium Pantothenate
☑ Delactosed Whey (pure whey safe; altered versions may contain gluten)
⊗ Della Rice (see page 24)
☑ Demineralized Whey (pure whey safe; altered versions may contain gluten)
☑ Desamidocollagen
☑ Dextran
? Dextrate (may be from any starch)
? Dextri-maltose (wheat barley may be used)
? Dextrin (can be made from wheat, corn, or several other grains; *supposed* to be indicated when wheat)
☑ Dextrose
☑ Dhal

☑Dhalin
☑Dichloromethane
☑Diglyceride (unmodified)
☑Dimethylpolysiloxane Formulations
⊗Dinkle (Spelt)
☑Dioctyl Sodium
☑Dioctyl Sodium Solfosuccinate
☑Dipotassium Phosphate
☑Disodium EDTA
☑Disodium Guanylate
☑Disodium Inosinate
☑Disodium Phosphate
⊗Disodium Wheatgermamido Peg-2 Sulfosuccinate
☑Distilled Alcohol (distillation process makes it safe; caution with added flavors, additives, color)
☑Distilled Vinegar (see "vinegar")
☑Dry Roasted Nuts (risk of cross contamination and seasoning)
⊗Durum Wheat (Triticum durum)
☑Dutch Processed Cocoa
?Edible Coatings/Films (may be corn or wheat)
⊗Edible Starch
☑EDTA (ethylenediaminetetraacetic acid)
☑Eggs
⊗Einkorn (Triticum monococcum)
☑Elastin
⊗Emmer (Triticum dicoccon)
⊗Emulsifiers (most contain gluten)
⊗Enriched Flour
⊗Enzymes (may contain binders)
☑Epichlorohydrin
☑Ergocalciferol
☑Erthorbic Acid

☑Erythritol
☑Erythrosine
☑Ester Gum
☑Ethanol
☑Ethoxyquin
☑Ethyl Alcohol
☑Ethylenediaminetetraacetic Acid
☑Ethyl Maltol
☑Ethyl Vanillin
☑Expeller Pressed Canola Oil (see Canola)
⊗Farina
⊗Farina Graham
⊗Farro
☑Fava Bean
☑Fennel
☑Ferric Orthophosphate
☑Ferrous Fumerate
☑Ferrous Gluconate
☑Ferrous Lactate
☑Ferrous Sulfate
☑Feta Cheese
⊗Filler (too vague, usually wheat)
☑Fish (caution with breaded, pre-seasoned, fried)
⊗Flaked Rice (see page 24)
?Flavoring (vague term)
☑Flax
⊗Flour (standard is wheat)
☑Flour Salt
☑Folacin
☑Folate
☑Folic Acid
?Food Coloring (vague)
?Food Starch (can be wheat or mixture)

☑Formaldehyde (gluten free, but toxic)
☑Fructose
☑Fructose Syrup (unflavored, for corn/corn fructose see page 24)
☑Fruit (if dried, verify for additives)
☑Fruit Juice Concentrate
☑Fruit Vinegar
⊗Fu (dried wheat gluten)
☑Fumaric Acid
☑Furcelleran
☑Galactose
?Gamma Oryzanol (verify starch used)
☑Garbanzo Beans
☑Garlic
☑Gelatin
?Gelatinized Starch (verify type of starch)
☑Gellan Gum
⊗Germ
⊗German Wheat
⊗Gliadin
☑Glucanase
☑Glucoamylase
☑Gluconic Acid
☑Glucono Lactone (Glucono-Delta)
☑Glucose
☑Glucose Isomerase
☑Glucose Oxidase
?Glucose Syrup (can be corn or wheat; usually listed as safe because the wheat forms are trace amounts. regardless of PPM level, *any* amount of gluten is not safe for a Celiac)
☑Glutamate

? Glutamic Acid (MSG, can be from several grains)
? Glutamine - glutamine & L-glutamine are the same: SAFE if the source is from animal protein or vegetable; UNSAFE when derived from wheat, peptide or bonded
⊗ Glutamine Peptide (usually derived from wheat)
⊗ Gluten
⊗ Glutenin
⊗ Gluten Peptides
⊗ Glutinous Rice   (see page 24)
? Glycerides (modified versions may contain wheat, unmodified are just fats and are safe)
☑ Glycerin
☑ Glycerol Diacetate
☑ Glycerol Monoacetate
☑ Glycerol Monooleate
☑ Glyceryl Triacetate
☑ Glyceryl Tributyrate
☑ Glycine
☑ Glycol
☑ Glycolic Acid
☑ Glycol Monosterate
⊗ Gorgonzola Cheese
⊗ Graham Flour
☑ Gram flour (chick peas)
⊗ Granary Flour (may be combination of grains)
☑ Grape Skin Extract
? Gravy (usually thickened with wheat flour, can be safe if pure corn starch)
⊗ Grits (corn – see page 24)
⊗ Groats (barley, wheat)
? Ground Spices (cross contamination/filler risk)
☑ Guaiaca Gum
☑ Guar Gum (guaran, can have IBS effect)
☑ Gum Acacia

☑Gum Arabic

?Gum Base (manufacturer must confirm source)

☑Gum Benzoin

☑Gum Guaiacum

☑Gum Tragacanth

⊗Hard Wheat

⊗Heeng

☑Hemicellulase

⊗Hemp (often listed as gluten free, but has been tested with 15 ppm gliadin)

☑Herbs (look for pure, many have fillers)

☑Herb Vinegar

☑Hexane

☑Hexanedioic Acid

⊗High Fructose Corn Syrup (see page 24)

⊗Hing

☑Hominy

☑Honey

☑Hops

⊗Hordein

⊗Hordeum Vulgare Extract

☑Horseradish (pure)

⊗HPP

?Hulls (outer layer of any grain)

⊗HVP

☑Hyacinth Bean

☑Hydrochloric Acid

⊗Hydrogenated Corn Starch

⊗Hydrogenated Starch Hydrolysate

☑Hydrogenated Vegetable Oil

☑Hydrogen Peroxide

☑Hydrolyzed Caseinate

☑Hydrolyzed Meat Protein

? Hydrolyzed Oat Protein (may contain wheat)
? Hydrolyzed Plant Protein (may contain wheat)
☑ Hydrolyzed Soy Protein
? Hydrolyzed Vegetable Protein (may contain wheat)
⊗ Hydrolyzed Wheat Gluten
⊗ Hydrolyzed Wheat Protein Pg-Propyl Silanetriol
⊗ Hydrolyzed Wheat Starch
☑ Hydroxylated Lecithin
☑ Hydroxypropyl Cellulose
☑ Hydroxypropyl Methylcellulose
⊗ Hydroxypropyltrimonium Hydrolyzed Wheat Protein
☑ Hypromellose
? Ice Cream (check ingredients, most have gluten)
⊗ Ice Cream Cones
☑ Illepe
☑ Indian Ricegrass seed (Montina)
☑ Indigotine
☑ Inulin
☑ Inulinase
☑ Invertase
☑ Invert Sugar
☑ Iodine
☑ Irish Moss Gelose
☑ Iron Ammonium Citrate
☑ Iron Oxide
☑ Isinglass
☑ Iso-Ascorbic Acid
☑ Isobutane
☑ Isolated Soy Protein
☑ Isomalt
☑ Isopropanol
☑ Isopropyl Alcohol
⊗ Japonica Rice (see page 24)

⊗ Jasmine Rice (see page 24)
☑ Job's Tears (Hato Mugi, Juno's Tears, River Grain)
⊗ Jowar (Sorghum, see page 24)
⊗ Kafirin
⊗ Kamut (pasta wheat)
☑ Karaya Gum
☑ Kasha (Russian Kasha may contain millet and oats)
☑ K-Carmine Color
⊗ Kecap Manis (soy sauce)
☑ Kelp
☑ Keratin
☑ Ketchup (check ingredients, many unsafe)
⊗ Ketjap Manis (soy sauce)
☑ K-Gelatin
⊗ Kluski Pasta
? Koji (verify starch used)
☑ Konjac
⊗ Koshihikari (rice – see page 24)
☑ Kudzu
☑ Kudzu Root Starch
☑ Lactalbumin Phosphate
☑ Lactase
☑ Lactic Acid
☑ Lactitol
☑ Lactobacillus Acidophilus
☑ Lactobacillus Bifidus
⊗ Lacto globulin
☑ Lactose (many Celiacs intolerant; reaction generally improves after adhering to GF diet for some time)
☑ Lactulose
☑ Lactylic Esters of fatty acids
☑ Lanolin

☑Lard
☑L-Cysteine
☑Lecithin (soy sensitive for some Celiacs)
☑Lecithin Citrate
☑Legumes
☑Lemon Grass
☑Lentils (careful with cross-contamination)
?L-Glutamine (see glutamine)
☑Licorice Candy or Extract (check with manufacturer)
☑Lipase
☑Lipoxidase
?Liquor (see alcohol)
☑L-Leucine
☑L-Lysine
☑L-Methionine
☑Locust Bean Gum
☑L-Tryptophan
☑Lysozyme
⊗Macha Wheat (triticum aestivum)
☑Magnesium Aluminum Silicate
☑Magnesium Carbonate
☑Magnesium Chloride
☑Magnesium Citrate
☑Magnesium Fumerate
☑Magnesium Hydroxide
☑Magnesium Oxide
☑Magnesium Phosphate
☑Magnesium Silicate
☑Magnesium Stearate
☑Magnesium Sulphate
⊗Maida (Indian wheat flour)
⊗Maize (corn – see page 24)

⊗Maize Waxy
☑Malic Acid
⊗Malt
⊗Malt Chocolate
⊗Malted Barley Flour
⊗Malted Milk
⊗Malt Extract
⊗Malt Flavoring
⊗Maltitol (usually listed as safe because process is supposed to remove gluten from the wheat starch – trace amounts will always be left)
?Maltodextrin (can be made from wheat, potato, rice or corn. listed as safe on most GF lists because it is a highly processed product, so assumption is gluten is removed even with wheat versions, but trace amounts may be left on product; not safe unless potato)
☑Maltol
⊗Maltose (listed as safe on most lists because the manufacturing process is said to remove the gluten from end product; trace amounts or more may be left)
⊗Malt Syrup
⊗Malt Vinegar
☑Manganese Sulfate
☑Manioc
☑Mannitol
☑Maple Syrup (pure, unflavored)
☑Margarine (check all ingredients)
⊗Masa Farina (cornstarch)
⊗Masa Flour
⊗Masa Harina
⊗Matza
⊗Matzah
⊗Matzo
⊗Matzo Semolina

☑Meat (watch for fillers, flavoring)

☑Medium Chain Triglycerides

☑Menhaden Oil

⊗Meringue

⊗Meripro 711

☑Methanol

☑Methyl Alcohol

☑Methyl Cellulose

☑Methyl Paraben

☑Microcrystalline Cellulose

☑Micro-Particulated Egg White Protein

☑Milk (technically safe, but many Celiacs sensitive – see "lactose". Caution if flavored; malted milk not safe)

☑Milk Protein Isolate (see milk or lactose)

⊗Millet (see page 24)

⊗Milo (Sorghum)

☑Mineral Oil

☑Mineral Salts

⊗Mir

⊗Mirin (many brands contain wheat)

⊗Miso

⊗Modified Corn Starch (see page 24)

?Modified Food Starch (caution, vague term)

☑Molasses (unflavored)

☑Molybdenum Amino Acid Chelate

☑Monoacetin (gluten free, food additive, also used as gelatinizing agent in explosives and leather tanning)

☑Monocalcium Phosphate

☑Monoglyceride (unmodified)

☑Monoisopropyl Citrate

☑Monopotassium Phosphate

☑Monosaccharides

? Monosodium Glutamate (see MSG)

☑Monostearates

? MSG (can be made from seaweed, wheat, or corn; always side with caution)

☑Mung Bean

☑Musk

☑Mustard powder or sauce (verify all ingredients)

☑Myristic Acid

☑Natamycin

? Natural Flavors (vague)

? Natural Juices (vague)

☑Natural Smoke Flavor

☑Neotame (gluten free, but toxic)

☑Niacin

☑Niacinamide

⊗Nishasta

☑Nitrates

☑Nitric Acid

☑Nitrogen

☑Nitrous Oxide

☑Non-fat Milk (unflavored, check additives)

☑Nori

☑Nuts (watch for risk of cross contamination in the roasting process and seasonings)

⊗Oat, Oatmeal, Oatrim (see page 24)

☑Oleic Acid

☑Oleoresin

☑Olestra (brand name Olean, gluten free, but a very harmful product found in many potato chips)

☑Oleyl Alcohol/Oil

☑Olive Oil

☑Orange B

☑Orchil

⊗Oriental Wheat (triticum turanicum)

⊗Oryzanol (usually rice bran oil, corn or barley)

⊗Orzenin (see page 24)

⊗Orzo Pasta

☑Oxystearin

☑Ozone

☑Palmitate

☑Palmitic Acid

☑Palm Kernel Oil (gluten free, but coconut oil is more environmentally friendly)

⊗Panicin (see page 24)

☑Pancreatin

☑Pantothenic Acid

☑Papain

☑Paprika

☑Paraffin

⊗Pasta (standard is wheat)

☑Pea - Chick

☑Pea - Cow

☑Pea Flour

☑Peanut (caution with roasted or seasoned)

☑Peanut Flour

☑Peanut Oil

⊗Pearl Barley

⊗Pearl Rice

☑Peas

☑Pea Starch

☑Pectin

☑Pectinase

☑Pentosanase

☑Peppermint Oil

☑Peppers
☑Pepsin
⊗Peptide Bonded Glutamine (usually wheat)
☑Peracetic Acid
⊗Persian Wheat (triticum carthlicum)
☑Peru Balsam
⊗Perungayam
☑Petrolatum
☑PGPR (Polyglycerol Polyricinoleate)
☑Phenylalanine
☑Phosphate (Calcium)
☑Phosphoric Acid
☑Phosphoric Glycol
☑Phosphorus Oxychloride
☑Pigeon Peas
☑Poi
⊗Polenta (corn – see page 24)
⊗Polished Rice
⊗Polish Wheat (triticum polonicum)
☑Polydextrose
☑Polyethylene Glycol
☑Polyglycerol
☑Polyglycerol Polyricinoleate (PGPR)
☑Polysorbates
⊗Popcorn (see page 24)
⊗Popcorn Rice (see page 24)
⊗Porter
☑Potassium Acid Tartrate
☑Potassium Benzoate
☑Potassium Bicarbonate
☑Potassium Bisulphite
☑Potassium Carbonate

☑Potassium Carrageenan
☑Potassium Caseinate
☑Potassium Citrate
☑Potassium Fumarate
☑Potassium Furcelleran
☑Potassium Hydroxide
☑Potassium Iodate
☑Potassium Iodide
☑Potassium Lactate
☑Potassium Matabisulphite
☑Potassium Nitrate
☑Potassium Phosphate
☑Potassium Sorbate
☑Potassium Stearate
☑Potassium Sulphate
☑Potassium Tartrate
☑Potato
?Potato Chips (look for specific GF products; usually unsafe due to seasonings and processing methods)
☑Potato Flour
☑Potato Starch
⊗Poulard Wheat (triticum turgidum)
☑Povidone
?Powdered Sugar (may contain gluten)
?Pregelatinized Starch (may be from any starch)
⊗Pretzels (many GF varieties available)
☑Prinus
☑Pristane
⊗Prolamin (see page 24)
☑Propionic Acid
☑Propolis
☑Propylene Glycol
☑Propylene Glycol Monosterate

☑Propyl Gallate
☑Protease
⊗Protein Hydrolysates
☑Psyllium
☑Pullulanase
☑Pyridoxine Hydrochloride
☑Pyrophosphate
☑Quinoa (risk of cross-contamination)
⊗Ragi (also called finger or African millet)
☑Raisin Vinegar
☑Rape (see Canola)
☑Recaldent
⊗Red Rice (see page 24)
☑Reduced Iron
☑Rennet
☑Rennet Casein
☑Resinous Glaze
☑Reticulin
☑Riboflavin
⊗Rice (see page 24)
⊗Rice Bran
⊗Rice Bran Oil
⊗Rice Flour
⊗Rice Malt (can also contain barley or Koji)
⊗Rice Milk
⊗Rice Paper
⊗Rice Polishings
⊗Rice Starch
⊗Rice Syrup (barley enzymes)
☑Rice Vinegar (check all ingredients, safe if distilled)
☑Ricinoleic Acid

⊗Risotto (Italian rice, see page 24)
☑Romano Bean (chickpea)
⊗Roquefort Cheese (listed as safe on most lists but usually contains trace amounts of gluten)
☑Rosematta
☑Rosin
⊗Rough Rice
⊗Roux (thickener, usually wheat flour)
☑Royal Jelly
⊗Rusk
⊗Rye
☑Saccharin
☑Safflower Oil (many Celiacs have reactions)
☑Saffron
☑Sago
☑Sago Flour or Starch
☑Sago Palm
☑Saifun (bean threads)
☑Salba
☑Salt
☑Saponin
?Sausage (check for fillers)
?Seasonings (caution with vague terms)
☑Seaweed (plain dry versions safe; caution with snack versions with added flavors like soy, which is unsafe)
⊗Secalin
⊗Seitan
⊗Semolina
⊗Semolina Triticum
☑Sesame
☑Sesame Butter (pure)
☑Shea
☑Sherry Vinegar

⊗Shortening (can contain vitamin E from wheat germ)
⊗Shot Wheat (triticum aestivum)
⊗Shoyu
☑Silicon Dioxide
⊗Sirimi (binder: usually wheat or cornstarch)
⊗Small Spelt
☑Soba (verify it is 100% buckwheat; also high risk of cross contamination)
☑Sodium Acetate
☑Sodium Acid Pyrophosphate
☑Sodium Alginate
☑Sodium Ascorbate
☑Sodium Benzoate
?Sodium Caseinate (contains MSG)
☑Sodium Citrate
☑Sodium Erythrobate
☑Sodium Hexametaphosphate
☑Sodium Lactate
☑Sodium Lauryl Sulfate (gluten free, but harmful product found in synthetic soap, shampoo, detergents – try to replace with phosphate free, natural products)
☑Sodium Metabisulphite
☑Sodium Nitrate
☑Sodium Phosphate
☑Sodium Polyphosphate
☑Sodium Silaco Aluminate
?Sodium Starch Glycolate (may be from any starch)
☑Sodium Stearoyl Lactylate
☑Sodium Sulphite
☑Sodium Stannate
☑Sodium Tripolyphosphate

⊗Soft Wheat
☑Sorbic Acid
☑Sorbitan Monostearate
☑Sorbitan Trioleate
☑Sorbitan Tristearate
☑Sorbitol-Mannitol (can cause IBS symptoms)
⊗Sorghum (see page 24)
⊗Sorgum (see page 24)
☑Soy (many Celiacs sensitive; soy sauce unsafe)
☑Soya Flour
☑Soya Starch
☑Soybean
☑Soy Lecithin
☑Soy Milk (check for added flavors or malt)
☑Soy Protein
☑Soy Protein Isolate
⊗Soy Sauce
⊗Spelt (triticum spelta)
☑Sphingolipids Soba (if it is 100% buckwheat)
?Spices (verify for fillers)
?Spirits (see alcohol)
⊗Sprouted Wheat or Barley
?Stabilizers (verify source)
?Starch (can be made from many sources)
⊗Stativa
☑Stearamide
☑Stearamine
☑Stearates
☑Stearic Acid
☑Stearyl Citrate
⊗Stearyldimoniumhydroxypropyl Hydrolyzed Wheat
Protein

☑ Stearyl Lactate
☑ Stevia
⊗ Stilton Cheese
⊗ Stock Cubes
⊗ Strong Flour
⊗ Stout
☑ Streptococcus Thermophilus
☑ Subflower Seed
☑ Succinic Anhydride
⊗ Succotash (corn and beans)
☑ Sucralose
☑ Sucrose
☑ Suet, raw fat safe (dried packet suet unsafe)
☑ Sugar (pure form, caution with powdered sugar)
☑ Sulfites
☑ Sulfosuccinate
☑ Sulfur Dioxide
☑ Sulphuric Acid
☑ Sulphurous Acid
☑ Sunflower oil or seed
⊗ Surimi
☑ Sweet Chestnut Flour
☑ Sweet Potato
⊗ Sweet Rice Flour
☑ Tagatose
☑ Tahini (100% pure sesame)
☑ Tallow
⊗ Tamari
☑ Tamarind
☑ Tannic Acid
☑ Tapioca
☑ Tapioca Flour

☑Tapioca Starch

☑Tara Gum

☑Taro

☑Tarro

☑Tarrow Root

☑Tartaric Acid

☑Tartrazine (gluten free, but harmful to health)

☑TBHQ - tertiary butylhydroquinone (gluten free preservative, but shown to be toxic in studies)

☑Tea (check for added ingredients)

☑Tea-Tree Oil

☑Teff (cross contamination risk)

?Tempeh (often contains soy sauce)

☑Tepary Bean

⊗Teriyaki Sauce

⊗Texmati Rice (see page 24)

?Textured Vegetable Protein (wheat or soy)

☑Thaumatin

☑Thiamine Hydrochloride

☑Thiamine Mononitrate

⊗Timopheevi Wheat (triticum timopheevii)

☑Titanium Dioxide

☑Tocopherols

☑Tofu (check for added ingredients)

☑Tolu Balsam

⊗Tortillas

☑Torula Yeast

⊗Tostada

☑Tragacanth

☑Tragacanth Gum

☑Triacetin

☑Tributyrin
☑Tricalcium Phosphate
☑Triethyl Citrate
⊗Triticale X Triticosecale
⊗Triticum Vulgare (wheat) Germ Extract or Oil
☑Trypsin
☑Turmeric
?TVP (can be wheat or soy)
☑Tyrosine
⊗Udon (usually wheat or corn)
⊗Unbleached Flour
☑Urad/Urid Beans
☑Urad/Urid Dal (peas) Vegetables
☑Urad/Urid flour
☑Urd
⊗Valencia Rice (see page 24)
☑Vanilla Extract (pure vanilla)
☑Vanilla Flavoring (verify it is pure vanilla)
☑Vanillin
⊗Vavilovi Wheat (triticum aestivum)
?Vegetable Broth
?Vegetable Gum (verify grains)
?Vegetable Protein
⊗Vegetable shortening
⊗Vegetable Starch (verify contents)
?Vinegar (apple cider, wine, or balsamic are usually safe; highly varied processes in making vinegar, manufacturer must be contacted in each case despite most lists claiming distilled as safe - additives are often added after distillation process. very inexpensive white vinegar must be verified)
⊗Vital Wheat Gluten
⊗Vulgar
⊗Waxy Maize

⊗Wehani Rice (see page 24)

⊗Wheat, abyssinian hard triticum durum

⊗Wheat Amino Acids

⊗Wheat Bran

⊗Wheat Bran Extract

⊗Wheat Bulgur

⊗Wheat Durum Triticum

⊗Wheat Germ

⊗Wheat Germamidopropyldimonium Hydroxypropyl

⊗Wheat Germ Glycerides

⊗Wheat Germ Oil

☑Wheatgrass (grass portion is safe, the seeds are not; if cutting to juice, cut one cm away from seed)

⊗Wheat Nuts

⊗Wheat Protein

⊗Wheat Triticum Aestivum

⊗Wheat Triticum Monococcum

☑Whey (pure whey safe; modified versions may contain trace amounts of gluten)

☑Whey Protein Concentrate

☑Whey Protein Isolate

⊗White Grain Vinegar

⊗Whole-Meal Flour

⊗Whole Wheat Berries

⊗Whole Wheat Flour

⊗Wild Einkorn (triticum boeotictim)

⊗Wild Emmer (triticum dicoccoides)

⊗Wild Rice (see page 24)

☑Wine (standard wine is safe; wine coolers are not)

☑Wine Vinegar (safe, see vinegar)

☑Wood Smoke

⊗Worcestershire (usually contains barley)

☑Xanthophyll

? Xanthum Gum (can be made from wheat, soy, corn, or dairy)

☑ Xylanase

☑ Xylitol

☑ Yam

☑ Yam Flour

? Yeast (Autolyzed, Baker's, Nutritional, Torula safe; Brewer's not safe. often grown or dried on wheat flour, side with caution, buy specially marked GF versions)

☑ Yogurt (caution with added flavors, fruit, toppings; added muesli or granola unsafe)

⊗ Zein (see page 24)

☑ Zinc Oxide

☑ Zinc Sulfate

WE, THE CONSUMER

Please look out for petitions you can sign, or letters you can send to government to bring transparency to food labels. As consumers, we have a right to know what is in our food, including genetically modified foods.

These dangerous laws must be changed, and like all social change, it is only through pressure from the public that it can happen.

As consumers, we don't realize we are collectively the most powerful force in the world – on ALL issues, food and otherwise. With every dollar we spend, we create demand, which dictates supply. By being aware of our choices and buying accordingly, we can create change. Every dollar spent is a powerful vote.

from one celiac
to another...

you are not alone

This is addressed first because the more support we have in managing *any* difficult situation, the better we tend to handle it. Ask for help. Do not isolate yourself.

There is a huge Celiac Circle out there, and even right here, with the words you are reading on this very page at this very moment.

Think of everyone around you, who love you, and have given you their support as you work your way through this.

Perhaps this situation is simply an opportunity to recognize and appreciate how much love is all around you.

Support groups can be extremely helpful. If that is not for you, go online and read through some comments on Celiac forums. It can be comforting to know that there are so many people who know exactly what you are going through.

You'll also pick up ideas, recipes, and many forum members share local information on restaurants offering gluten free food, grocery stores and specialty shops that bring in GF products, and even feedback on specific gluten free products.

You are truly not alone.

purity

The gluten free diet is one of purity. It is a wonderful way for your body to rid itself of so much and allow you to taste foods in their natural form.

Enjoy the freshness of fruits and vegetables. Appreciate the flavor in a single grain of rice and the freshness of freshly squeezed orange juice.

There is no store bought dip in the world that can compete with the incredible taste of fresh guacamole. Ripe avocados, tomatoes, cilantro, freshly squeezed lime juice...all mixing together in rich greens and red. An absolute feast for eyes, smell, and taste!

I used to think lasagna was delicious. I thought I would really miss it. Then I realized the flavor doesn't really come from the noodle; it comes from the tomato sauce, spices, and cheese. Try making eggplant lasagna - be generous with the mozzarella, and throw on freshly chopped basil as you serve for added aroma. You'll wonder why you haven't been preparing it this way all along (and of course, gluten free noodles are also now available).

Ridding toxins in our body can sometimes help in getting rid of externally harmful conditions as well. Are there areas in your life that are causing you stress and causing your entire being to be at dis-ease? It may be time to take a step back and make some positive changes, not just with your diet.

Look for new and exotic fruits, spices, and vegetables. Who can resist the colorful spices of Morocco, India, Thailand? Not appealing to you? How about Mexican corn tacos, Southwestern chili peppers, grilled Hawaiian pineapple?

Discover new parts of your own city. How much time have you actually spent roaming around Little Italy, Chinatown, Latin Quarter, Greek Quarter?

You will usually find people to be extremely friendly and helpful. They are so pleased and proud to introduce their food and culture to you. You might make friendships you never imagined.

If you live in a city that doesn't have ethnic quarters, you still have plenty of avenues you can take. Cookbooks from around the world that will show you how to make things you have never heard of or online stores that can ship fantastic spices to you. How about a weekend getaway to the town next door that has some interesting shops?

Enroll in an un-cooking class (raw food), perhaps get a friend or significant other to take the class with you, and then throw a food party! Try a chip & dip party with a variety of tapenades and homemade raw dips.

You have a whole world to explore, right in your own city and grocery store. So exciting!

show your colors

We as human beings are really so strong and resilient. YOU are stronger than you can ever imagine and can handle anything that comes your way.

Approach it in steps:
- gather knowledge - you can't win at a game you don't understand
- reorganize your diet – immediately get rid of what is harmful, and then slowly build up a new diet of safe foods
- get support – everything is easier to manage when we do it with help
- stay informed – there are always new products and new information coming out
- create a plan to build back your health – make it your priority, is there anything more important than your health?

But most importantly, make the whole process of changing your diet a fun thing. I am not making light of a serious condition: before being diagnosed I spent months enduring excruciating cramps and suffering from severe dehydration.

In life, it doesn't really matter what experiences are thrown on your path; what matters is your reaction to them. The same experience, no matter what it is, can have both a negative and positive outcome. Attitude is everything.

So, how will *you* decide to handle this?

Your body has given you a signal that it needs change. If you are like me, there were several lighter signals long before the major symptoms surfaced. I didn't listen and kept going 100 miles an hour until I had no option. A deeper connection with your body will help you help yourself.

What level of stress are you forcing your mind and body to endure? Are you doing anything to counter that stress? Find a way to have some time, *ANY* time, to yourself each day. It can be a 5 minute meditation just before bed or in the am before the day starts – begin there, and work on increasing time for yourself.

Even if you already work out, consider something new that helps connect mind and body. Try yoga by Shiva Rea; she has an incredible style that gives you so much more than exercise. She has several DVD's available on Amazon, each better than the next.

DVDs are great! Being able to practice at home makes it so convenient; you can take it at your own pace and work it into your schedule no matter how hectic.

Connecting with nature also always helps us connect with ourselves. A weekend in the country might do you wonders. Hiking, kayaking, beachcombing – it doesn't need to be strenuous, it just needs to resonate well with you and make you feel good. For some people feeling good means peaceful relaxation with a good book and for others it's exhilaration.

break from celiac

It's easy to become consumed with something that affects you every day; however it is important for your mental and emotional well being for you to not become the disease and nothing else.

Prepare several meals ahead of time and forget your Celiac state for a few days. Certainly, you need to be conscious of everything you eat and drink – but it can't become everything you are and it can't take over your life. When I was first diagnosed, meals became so stressful – and I quickly realized it wasn't a good idea to deal with this morning, noon, and night every day. So I spent a little extra time prepping on Sundays, and again in the middle of the week. There you have it, Celiac only took away a few hours from me twice a week until I was completely used to it. Much easier.

I've also enrolled friends to take care of my food for a weekend away together. OF COURSE make sure they are well versed with gluten restrictions, that they are using a safe/unsafe list for any products used in the meal preparation, or that they are enrolling on a raw food weekend that is safe for you and a detox weekend for them! I've done this with friends and family, and in exchange for their food efforts I was in charge of all drinks.

For your mental and emotional well being, take conscious vacations away from Celiac and soon you will find yourself not noticing the difference between the two worlds.

take it easy

Go easy on yourself. There is a lot to process; you cannot expect to gather masses of information overnight. Start with what is critical and immediately eliminate from your diet what can harm you. Then slowly reorganize your kitchen. Know that it will all get done, and take it step by step.

With the right outlook, new foods or different ways of cooking your old ones can be fun to do. Don't allow your new diet to feel like a constraint, but see it as a new exploration.

Choose relaxed days like Sundays to find and experiment with new recipes, get enjoyment from it! Remember this is an ongoing process and it will be unnecessarily more difficult if you put pressure on yourself.

Prioritize and do things in a relaxed pace. After all, much of the research so far is showing us that stress plays a major role in triggering Celiac in the first place. The last thing we need to do is stunt our own healing by making the healing process itself stressful.

We are all slowly starting to learn that the effects of stress are much more serious than we ever thought. Learn how to minimize the stress you are feeling and try to find activities that will help counter the stress you encounter day to day. A 20 minute walk after work might do wonders to press your restart button. Try parking 5 blocks away and look forward to that decompression time before the next task.

healing foods

Do some research on foods that will help your healing and contribute to your good health. Discover new ingredients, or old ones you never realized were good for you (make sure to keep a running list).

Example: ginger is a natural anti-inflammatory. Peel, cut, and boil pieces to make tea. Warm or iced, add some lemon and honey – it's fabulous!

When I was first diagnosed, my intestines had suffered extensive damage. Aloe Vera juice helps to heal intestines, but it tastes horrible. So every day I'd shake up 2oz of Aloe Vera juice with 4oz of pure grape or cranberry juice and serve it in a martini glass.

My daily cocktail not only facilitated a speedy recovery, it began a spectacular habit of having some down time before putting dinner together. Thankfully, I don't need the Aloe Vera anymore, but I very rarely miss my luxurious evening cocktail which is now a fruit smoothie packed with vitamins and antioxidants...still served in a martini glass...

B vitamins are important for a healthy gastrointestinal tract and they are in so many foods: nuts and vegetables high in protein, cheese, eggs, fish, meat, raisins, peanut butter (peanut butter cookies count!).

Chocolate contains powerful antioxidants - that one's easy to love!

hydration

Dehydration is a problem for most Celiacs, particularly in the beginning, when your intestines are not absorbing food or water very well. For everyone, water is vital, but for us it is even more important to drink more water than usual.

This might be easier to do if you make it more interesting in a natural way. Using a glass pitcher or carafe, add slices of citrus – lemon/lime if you like sour, orange if you prefer sweet. Try fresh or frozen raspberries, strawberries, or blackberries - it looks gorgeous and tastes fabulous. Cinnamon sticks, mint leaves, virtually any flavor you like will make it a lot easier to drink plenty of water.

I'd encourage you to turn to nature to flavor your water. There are an unprecedented number of flavored waters on the market now; besides being a gluten risk due to the coloring, it really isn't good for the body to process synthetic beverages or even food for that matter. The first and most important item in our diets that should remain pure is water.

Another trick is to get a glass you love. Go out and shop for a special one. I drink water from a big round crystal wine goblet. I love how it feels in my hand and reflects light when the sun touches it. Along with a tall sculpture-like carafe, it's a much more pleasurable experience and don't we all do more of things when we enjoy them?

upgrade

Now that we are eliminating harmful things from our diet and making fantastic improvements, it's the perfect time to upgrade on a few things.

Toss out the old salt and pepper shakers and get terrific new grinders with flavorful fresh peppercorns and pure Himalayan salt.

If you're a coffee drinker, get a grinder and try out blends from around the world (fair trade please). Forget cream and sugar, drink it black and get the true taste of coffee. If you do that for a week, your palette will change and you won't want to drink coffee any other way.

Tea drinker? Find a tea house and buy whole leaf teas. I love orchid oolong or jasmine green tea. The health benefits are countless, as you are hearing & reading everywhere and the no-risk factor of whole leaf versus processed makes it an easy choice.

One of the best purchases you can make is a juicer. The newer models are pretty easy to clean up, but regardless of that, the benefits are well worth a little effort. Even if you are eating a fantastic diet, you cannot consume in a day, or even 5 days, the nutrients you will get from a glass of fresh carrots, celery, and apples. There is no way any of us would eat pounds of carrots, a full head of celery, and several apples every day; but that's what it takes to make a glass of juice. By far, a great way to feed your body goodness.

It may seem overwhelming to find substitutes for so many foods you are used to. You don't need to tackle it all at the same time.

A great trick is to choose one item a week – let's say bread this week (gluten free versions are usually in the frozen foods section), cereal next week (great GF granolas are available), etc.

Certainly, if you have the time, go ahead and explore aisle after aisle. But if you don't have those hours, don't let it get to you; every week, 5 minutes, one item, and before you know it, every ingredient in your refrigerator and pantry will be replaced.

Something I'd like to reiterate here: please do not rely on gluten free grocery end-product guides entirely. Manufacturers change their ingredients often; for your safety, make sure you are always checking all ingredients for store bought products.

You can also use the one-at-a-time trick to replace gluten in meals you enjoy. Choose a meal a week and figure out how to make it safe for you. Squash spaghetti instead of wheat is easy with a shredder. Melted pure chocolate, nuts, and honey to replace your regular granola bars; you make them once a week and they are ready to go snacks all week – not to mention packed with punch! Chocolate (pure) is a fantastic antioxidant, nuts are rich in protein and several vitamins, and honey is a natural energy booster.

family & friends

This can get tricky and sometimes even difficult.

It is important to explain to your close family and friends the details and severity of your food restrictions. I've been contaminated with undetectable traces of spices and then had to hear "it was only a pinch, for flavor". Clearly, I had not done a good job of explaining that one grain of gluten is an issue.

Many of us get uneasy here; we don't want to put anyone out of their way. The reality is, it doesn't have to be that much trouble. In the case of a salad, a plate just needs to be set aside before any regular dressing is mixed in. Then that plate can get flavored with lemon, olive oil, salt, pepper and you are safe. That would not take more than 30 seconds.

Meat, chicken, or fish: a portion simply needs to be set aside for you and flavored with just salt, pepper, olive oil. If cooking on a grill, your portion gets cooked first, before the grill is contaminated, and then everyone else's can follow; if oven, cook separately in aluminum foil. It really is easy.

It comes down to communication and it usually doesn't need to be more than once. If you become reserved about the topic and don't properly explain it to people around you, this is where you will run into trouble. Take the time, make sure everyone understands, at least to some degree, what Celiac is and how harmful gluten is to you.

remain steadfast

Remember that Celiac is not a disease that is understood by the general public yet. Do not allow anyone to pressure you into eating something that you know is harmful.

"But it's your Dad's birthday! Just a little piece of cake won't kill you..."

Yes. It will. Or at least it will set you back for no reason.

Your health is completely & solely your responsibility.

You are the one that will suffer the consequences; you need to be the one to make sure you remain safe.

Understand that people will be uncomfortable if they are eating something and you are not; they care for you and don't want you to feel left out – their intentions are good. Sometimes they simply feel like they are being bad hosts if a guest is unable to eat foods served, it is up to you to reassure them.

They simply don't understand the disease and it will be up to you to remain steadfast and make sure you are not inflicting damage on yourself. Sometimes you might not want to go into details, especially with unfamiliar people. You don't have to. Just say no thanks and stick with it. I've been to several parties filled with strangers, heard "watching your waist?" every time I declined a food, and simply responded "yes, something like that". It's as simple as that.

celiac and depression

This subject is vast enough to warrant volumes of books on its own, so please don't consider this minuscule touch on the matter as anything more than a slight indication letting you know that if you haven't been feeling like yourself, there are probably chemical reasons why.

Celiac and depression are related. The reason for this is simple: Celiac causes malabsorption in the body and one of the main factors causing depression is vitamin and mineral deficiency, creating physical imbalance.

As of 2009, studies from patients diagnosed with Celiac are showing it takes an average of 11 years before most Celiacs are correctly diagnosed. ELEVEN years or more of the body slowly being drained of essential vitamins and minerals...

...combined with generally poor diets, contaminants in food, air, water, life stresses from work and personal lives...   The human body can only take so much.

Depression is a mental breakdown. Literally. It is a lack of essential fatty acids and vitamins to the brain causing neurotransmitters (the brain's messengers) to malfunction or completely disconnect and stop functioning. This is what makes a person's serotonin (happy mood) level drop, melatonin (help to sleep) level drop, and much more – causing a severe imbalance - which leads to depression and worse. Depression IS treatable; but you need to restore your body with everything it has become depleted of.

These may help restore your balance:

-B Complex (a superior B Complex will include 100mg B6, 100mcg B12, as well as folic acid)

-Folic Acid 1mg

-Magnesium, 300mg

-Vitamin D, 1000 I.U.

-DHA/EPA (preferably in liquid form) 2500-3000mg

-Flax Seed Oil, 1000mg/day

(All these dosages are general guidelines, please see pages 20-21 regarding dosages)

Your body has slowly been depleted of vital vitamins; so slowly, you probably never even noticed the changes happening until one day you woke up realizing how low you feel. *We must stop seeing depression as a condition and recognize is as current health status.*

Understand the importance of fatty acids: the brain is made up 60% of fat, half of that is DHA (omega 3). Why am I not suggesting you just take omega 3's? Because you need a perfect ratio of omega 3 and 6 to form DHA, which is what your brain really needs. Instead of becoming a mad scientist and trying to figure out what that balance is, you can just buy DHA.

Flax seeds contain a lot of omega 3 as well, but can be a little delicate to handle. The oil loses potency with light, the ground seeds lose potency to air – it needs to be consumed immediately after being ground.

I sincerely believe in holistic remedies whenever possible; though certainly sometimes the situation can get grave enough to warrant prescription medication – try to make that an absolute last resort.

Try to exhaust all natural remedies before going the prescription route. Most of the time, solutions can be found in nature, sustainable long term, and with no side effects. Meaning even herbal remedies (listed below) should not be needed for a lifetime once the body is properly nourished. Until that point, here are two effective ones you can try:

SAMe – depression comes from deficiencies of certain chemicals in the brain; SAMe is an amino acid that your brain needs to maintain healthy neurotransmitter processes.

5-HTP – also an amino acid. The tryptophan in 5-HTP also helps your body naturally generate melatonin, which helps maintain regular sleep patterns. Usually effective, though it leaves some people feeling tired the next morning.

There are several others you can try, though I have not found them to be as safe as SAMe and 5-HTP.

Exercise naturally increases your body's own anti-stress hormones. Scientists can directly connect exercise with increased efficiency of neurotransmitters in the brain to help alleviate depression.

Any method is good: yoga, walking, jogging, dance, swimming, weights, cycling... Whatever type of exercise you can do, at least 3-4 times a week for a minimum of 30 minutes will help. Needless to say, daily is best.

Modern medicine also keeps proving that positive feelings like love and gratitude naturally increase the DHEA levels in your body. A cruel catch 22 – how do you force happiness in order to achieve happiness? Try a gratitude journal: spend 5 minutes a day focused on the blessings in your life. Seeing how much you are blessed with should make you feel really good for those 5 minutes, and soon they will become 20, 60, and then all the time.

If you can't seem to escape from thoughts of hopelessness or worse, PLEASE get help. You are fighting a very serious chemical war inside yourself, and this is not something that you should fight alone. THIS STATE IS NOT YOU. What you are feeling is not the real you, and there is definitely a solution.

The suggestions and guidelines in the previous pages will help the majority of people suffering from depression. However in some cases, the physical damage might be too extensive to be self-cured. In some cases, the length of time the body has been deteriorating has been too long and the person might need to work with a doctor or naturopath to bring balance back.

Please get qualified help. There IS a way out of this dark maze you feel like you are trapped in; and like all mazes, it is a lot easier for someone from the outside to see the exits than the person in the maze.

You deserve, as everyone does, to live a happy and fulfilled life. Please do not suffer needlessly and do not give up. Just take a little leap of faith that there is a solution out there for you and ask for help. You can be well once again, just a tiny leap of faith...

notes

notes

notes

notes

notes

notes

notes

notes

notes

notes

notes

notes

notes

notes

notes

notes

notes

ESSENTIAL BASICS PAGE INDEX

COPYRIGHT © 2011 BLACK WAVE PUBLISHING

ALL RIGHTS RESERVED. REPRODUCTION IN ANY MANNER WITHOUT WRITTEN PERMISSION IS PROHIBITED, EXCEPT FOR BRIEF QUOTATIONS USED IN CONNECTION WITH MEDIA REVIEWS.

PRINTED IN THE UNITED STATES

LIBRARY AND ARCHIVES CANADA

KARR, JAQUI.
      CELIAC DISEASE: SAFE/UNSAFE FOOD LIST AND ESSENTIAL INFORMATION ON LIVING WITH A GLUTEN FREE DIET

ISBN: 978-0-9813198-7-2

3RD REVISION

15787622R00051

Made in the USA
Lexington, KY
16 June 2012